The Complete Mediterranean Cookbook

Heal your body with the ultimate collection of easy and tasty Mediterranean recipes

Carlo Montesanti

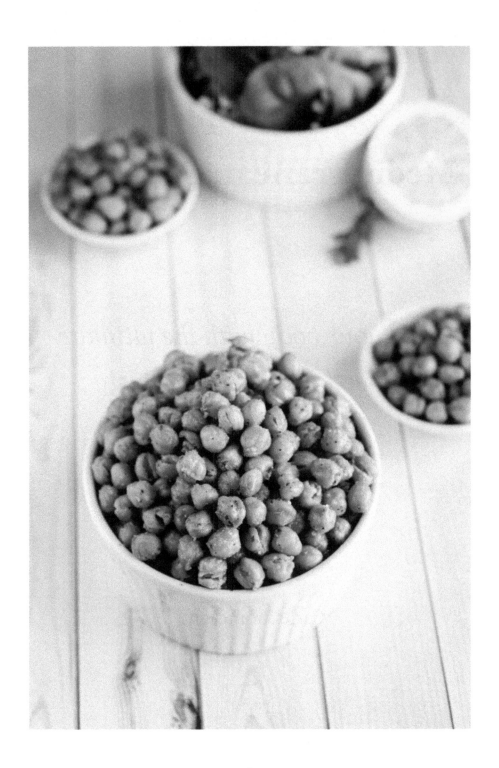

implied. readers acknowledge that the author is not engaging in the rendering of legal, financial, medical or professional advice. the content within this book has been derived from various sources. please consult a licensed professional before attempting any techniques outlined in this book.

by reading this document, the reader agrees that under no circumstances is the author responsible for any losses, direct or indirect, which are incurred as a result of the use of information contained within this document, including, but not limited to, — errors, omissions, or inaccuracies.

Table of Contents

Cauliflower Fritters

Prep Time: 10 min

Cook Time: 50 min

Serve: 4

Ingredients:

- 30 oz. canned chickpeas, drained and rinsed

- 2 and ½ tbsp. olive oil

- 1 small yellow onion, chopped

- 2 cups cauliflower florets chopped

- 2 tbsp. garlic, minced

- A pinch of salt and black pepper

Preparation:

1. Spread half of the chickpeas on a baking sheet lined with parchment pepper, add 1 tbsp. oil, season with salt and pepper, toss and bake at 400°F for 30 minutes.

2. Transfer the chickpeas to a food processor, pulse well and put the mix into a bowl.

3. Heat a pan with the ½ tbsp. oil over medium-high heat, add the garlic and the onion and sauté for 3 minutes.

4. Add the cauliflower, cook for 6 minutes more, transfer this to a blender, add the rest of the chickpeas, pulse, pour over the crispy chickpeas mix from the bowl, stir and shape medium patties out of this mix. Heat a pan with the rest of the oil over medium-high heat, add the patties, cook them for 3 minutes on each side, and serve breakfast.

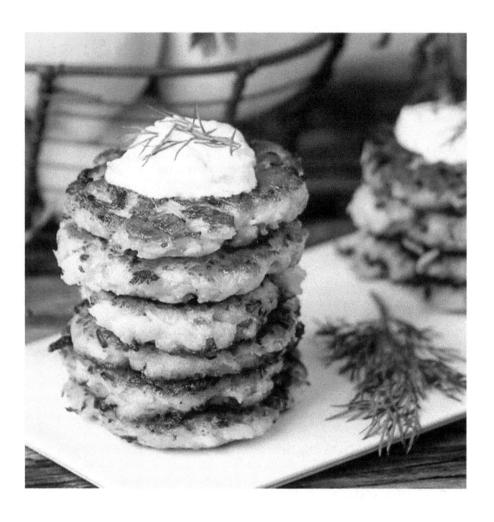

Mediterranean Chickpea Snack

Prep Time: 30 min

Cook Time: 0 min

Serve: 2

Ingredients:

- ½ tsp. garlic powder

- 1 can (10 oz.) chickpeas, rinsed and drained

- ½ tsp. dried basil

- 1 tsp. extra-virgin olive oil

- ¼ tsp. sea salt

- 1 tsp. Nutritional Yeast

- ¼ tsp. red pepper flakes

Preparation:

1. Preheat the oven to 450°F. Line a baking pan with a parchment paper. Grease it with some refined coconut oil or avocado oil (You can also use cooking spray). Combine the chickpeas, seasonings, and oil in a mixing bowl.

2. Arrange the chickpeas in the pan. Roast the chickpeas for about 10 minutes. Toss and keep roasting for 10 more minutes. Serve warm.

Avocado Chickpea Pizza

Prep Time: 20 min

Cook Time: 20 min

Serve: 2

Ingredients:

- 1 and ¼ cups chickpea flour
- A pinch of salt and black pepper
- 1 and ¼ cups water
- 2 tbsp. olive oil
- 1 tsp. onion powder
- 1 tsp. garlic, minced
- 1 tomato, sliced
- 1 avocado, peeled, pitted and sliced
- 2 oz. gouda, sliced

- ¼ cup tomato sauce

- 2 tbsp. green onions, chopped

Preparation:

1. In a bowl, mix the chickpea flour with salt, pepper, water, the oil, onion powder and the garlic, stir well until you obtain a dough, knead a bit, put in a bowl, cover and leave aside for 20 minutes. Transfer the dough to a working surface, shape a bit circle, transfer it to a baking sheet lined with parchment paper and bake at 425°F for 10 minutes.

2. Spread the tomato sauce over the pizza, spread the rest of the ingredients and bake at 400°F for 10 minutes more.

3. Cut and serve for breakfast.

Pita Wedges with Almond Bean Dip

Prep Time: 10 min

Cook Time: 5 min

Serve: 5

Ingredients:

- 8 oz. beet, cubed

- 5 garlic cloves, peeled

- ¼ cup almond, slivered

- 15 ½ oz. garbanzo beans

- ¾ cup extra-virgin olive oil

- 1 ½ tbsp. red wine vinegar

- Whole-wheat pita wedges to serve

Preparation:

1. In a saucepan or deep skillet, boil the beet in sufficient water quantity until it is tender. Drain, peel, cut in cubes and blend in a food processor. Add the garbanzo beans, almonds, oil, and garlic and blend everything well until smooth. Add the red wine and blend for one more minute.

2. Season with black pepper and salt.

3. Chill in the refrigerator. Serve with pita wedges.

Ginger Antipasti

Prep Time: 10 min

Cook Time: 0 min

Serve: 6

Ingredients:

- 1 tsp. ginger powder

- 1 cup fresh parsley, chopped

- 1 tbsp. apple cider vinegar

- 3 tbsp. avocado oil

- 2 oz celery stalk, chopped

Preparation:

Mix all ingredients in the bowl and leave for 5 minutes in the fridge.

Mediterranean Chickpea Spread

Prep Time: 8 min

Cook Time: 5 min

Serve: 2

Ingredients:

- 2 cups chickpeas (canned or pre-soaked and cooked)
- 2 tbsp. lemon juice
- 1/2 tsp. cumin
- 2 cloves garlic, minced
- 4 tsp. olive oil
- Salt to taste
- Ground cinnamon (optional)

Preparation:

1. In a mixing bowl, add the chickpeas; mash thoroughly using a fork (you can also use a blender).

2. Add the olive oil, garlic and lemon juice. Combine well; top with some cinnamon. Serve with vegetable sticks, whole-wheat crackers, or whole-wheat pita wedges.

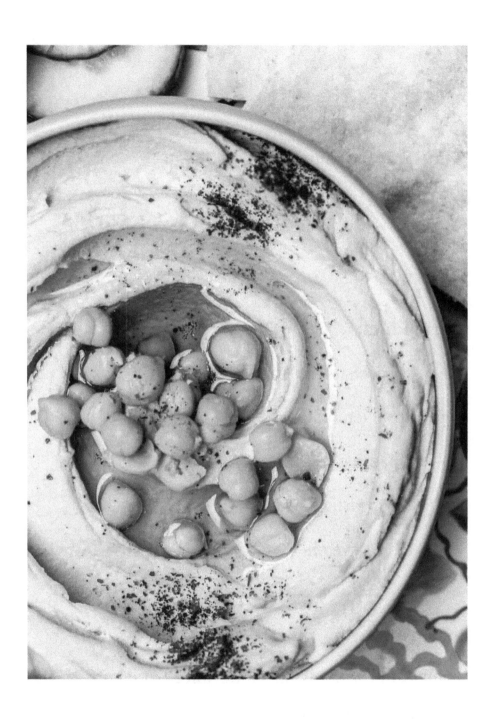

Rosemary Beets

Prep Time: 10 min

Cook Time: 4 min

Serve: 6

Ingredients:

- 1-lb. beets, sliced, peeled

- 2 tbsp. lemon juice

- 1 tsp. dried rosemary

- ¼ tsp. garlic powder

- 1 tbsp. olive oil

Preparation:

Sprinkle the beets with lemon juice, rosemary, garlic powder, and olive oil. Then preheat the grill to 400°F.

Place the sliced beet in the grill and cook it for 2 minutes per side.

Scallions Dip

Prep Time: 5 min

Cook Time: 15 min

Serve: 4

Ingredients:

- 1 cup spinach, chopped

- 2 oz scallions, chopped

- ¼ cup plain yogurt

- ¼ tsp. chili powder

- 1 tsp. olive oil

Preparation:

1. Melt the olive oil in the saucepan. Add spinach and scallions. Saute the greens for 10 minutes.

2. Then add chili powder and plain yogurt. Stir well and cook it for 5 minutes more. Then blend the mixture with the help of the immersion blender.

Dill Tapas

Prep Time: 5 min

Cook Time: 0 min

Serve: 8

Ingredients:

- ½ tsp. garlic powder

- 2 cups plain yogurt

- ½ cup dill, chopped

- ¼ tsp. ground black pepper

- 2 pecans, chopped

- 2 tbsp. lemon juice

Preparation:

Put all ingredients in the bowl and stir well with the help of the spoon.

Sour Cream Dip

Prep Time: 10 min

Cook Time: 0 min

Serve: 8

Ingredients:

- 4 oz yogurt

- ¼ tsp. chili flakes

- ¼ tsp. salt

- 2 avocados, peeled, pitted

- 1 tsp. olive oil

- ½ tsp. lemon juice

- 2 tbsp. fresh parsley, chopped

Preparation:

1. Put all ingredients in the blender and blend until smooth.

2. Store the dip in the closed vessel in the fridge for up to 5 days.

Arugula Antipasti

Prep Time: 5 min

Cook Time: 0 min

Serve: 8

Ingredients:

- 2 oz chives, chopped
- 1 cup arugula, chopped
- 2 cups chickpeas, canned
- 1 jalapeno pepper, chopped
- 1 tbsp. avocado oil
- 1 tsp. lemon juice

Preparation:

Put all ingredients in the bowl and stir well.

Goat Cheese Dip

Prep Time: 10 min

Cook Time: 8 min

Serve: 4

Ingredients:

- 3 oz goats cheese, soft
- 2 oz plain yogurt
- 2 oz chives, chopped
- 1 tbsp. lemon juice
- ¼ tsp. ground black pepper
- 2 bell peppers

Preparation:

1. Grill the bell peppers for 3-4 minutes per side.

2. Then peel the peppers and remove seeds.

3. Then put bell peppers in the blender. Add all remaining ingredients, blend them well and transfer in the ramekins.

Mozzarella Dip

Prep Time: 10 min

Cook Time: 20 min

Serve: 10

Ingredients:

- 1-lb. artichoke hearts, diced

- ¾ cup spinach, chopped

- 1 cup mozzarella cheese, grated

- 1 tsp. Italian seasonings

- ½ tsp. garlic powder

- ¼ cup organic almond milk

Preparation:

Put all ingredients in the saucepan, stir well, and close the lid. Saute the meal on low heat for 20 minutes. Stir it from time to time. Then chill the dip well.

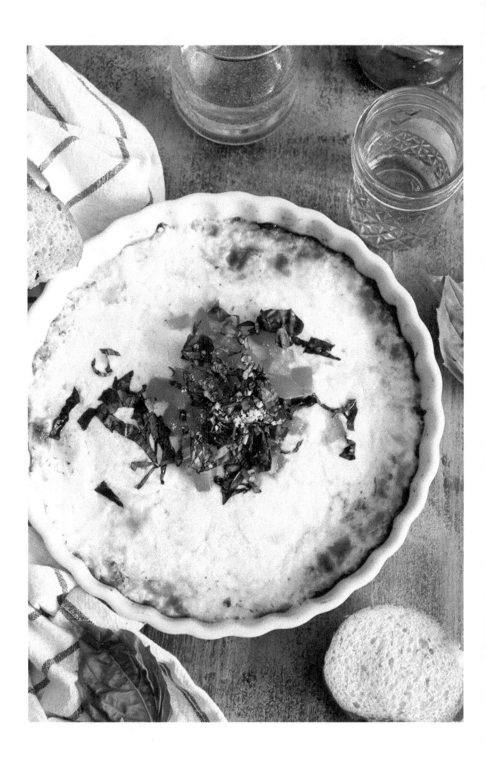

Spicy Salsa

Prep Time: 40 min

Cook Time: 0 min

Serve: 16

Ingredients:

- 3 cups tomatoes, chopped

- 1 tsp. salt

- 1 tsp. white pepper

- ½ cup red onion, chopped

- 1 cup fresh cilantro, chopped

- 1 jalapeno pepper, chopped 1 tbsp. olive oil

- 1 tbsp. apple cider vinegar

Preparation:

1. Put all ingredients in the salad bowl and mix well.

2. Leave the cooked salsa for 30 minutes in the fridge.

Cheese Spread

Prep Time: 10 min

Cook Time: 8 min

Serve: 6

Ingredients:

- ½ cup cream cheese

- 1 pickle, grated

- 1 oz fresh dill, chopped

- ¼ tsp. ground paprika

Preparation:

1. Carefully mix cream cheese with dill and ground paprika.

2. Then add a grated pickle and gently mix the spread.

Prosciutto Beans

Prep Time: 10 min

Cook Time: 0 min

Serve: 8

Ingredients:

- 2 cups canned cannellini beans, drained

- 1 tbsp. scallions, diced

- 3 tbsp. olive oil

- ¼ tsp. chili flakes 1 tbsp. lemon juice

- 3 oz beef, chopped, cooked

Preparation:

Put all ingredients in the bowl and stir well.

Carrot Chips

Prep Time: 5 min

Cook Time: 10 min

Serve: 6

Ingredients:

- 2 carrots, thinly sliced

- 1 tsp. salt

- 1 tsp. olive oil

Preparation:

1. Line the baking tray with baking paper. Then arrange the sliced carrot in one layer.

2. Sprinkle the vegetables with olive oil and salt. Bake the carrot chips for 10 minutes or until the vegetables are crunchy.

Antipasti Salad

Prep Time: 10 min

Cook Time: 0 min

Serve: 4

Ingredients:

- ½ cup green olives, pitted and sliced

- 1 cucumber, spiralized

- 1 cup cherry tomatoes, halved

- 4 oz Feta cheese, crumbled

- 2 tbsp. olive oil

Preparation:

1. Put green olives, spiralized cucumber, and cherry tomatoes in the bowl. Add olive oil and stir well.

2. Then top the salad with Feta.

Black Olives Spread

Prep Time: 10 min

Cook Time: 0 min

Serve: 10

Ingredients:

- 3 cups black olives, pitted

- ½ cup chickpeas, canned

- 1 tsp. Italian seasonings

- 3 tbsp. sunflower oil

- ½ tsp. ground black pepper

Preparation:

Put all ingredients in the blender and blend until smooth.

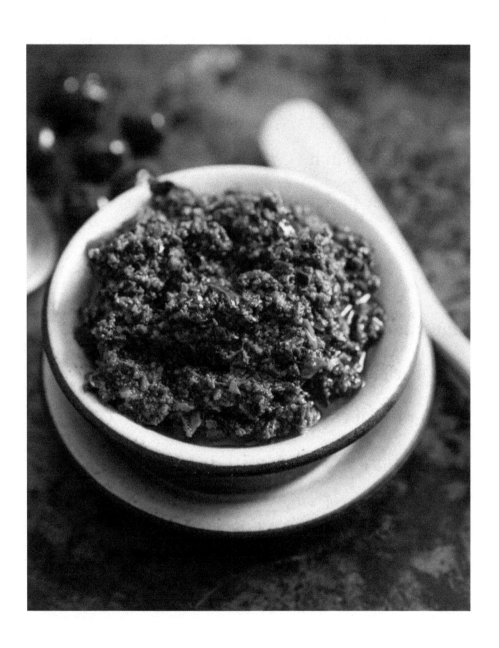

Bell Pepper Antipasti

Prep Time: 10 min

Cook Time: 4 min

Serve: 6

Ingredients:

- 5 bell peppers

- 1 tbsp. olive oil

- 3 tbsp. avocado oil

- ½ tsp. salt

- 2 garlic cloves, minced

- 3 tbsp. fresh cilantro, chopped

Preparation:

1. Pierce the bell peppers with the help of a knife and sprinkle with olive oil. Grill the vegetables at 400F for 2 minutes per side. Then peel them and remove seeds.

2. Put the grilled bell peppers in the blender and add all remaining ingredients. Blend the mixture well.

Hummus Rings

Prep Time: 10 min

Cook Time: 0 min

Serve: 4

Ingredients:

- ½ cup hummus
- 2 cucumbers

Preparation:

Roughly slice the cucumbers and remove the cucumber flesh. Then fill every cucumber ring with hummus.

Fish Strips

Prep Time: 10 min

Cook Time: 0 min

Serve: 4

Ingredients:

- 1 cucumber, sliced

- 1 tsp. apple cider vinegar

- 2 tbsp. plain yogurt

- 1 tsp. dried dill

- 3 oz salmon, smoked, sliced

Preparation:

1. Arrange the sliced cucumber in the plate in one layer.

2. Then sprinkle them with apple cider vinegar, plain yogurt, and dried dill.

3. Then top the cucumbers with sliced salmon.

Vegetable Balls

Prep Time: 10 min

Cook Time: 5 min

Serve: 8

Ingredients:

- 2 eggplants, grilled
- 2 tbsp. olive oil
- 1 garlic clove, minced
- 1 egg, beaten
- ½ cup oatmeal, ground
- ½ tsp. ground black pepper
- 2 oz Parmesan, grated

Preparation:

1. Blend the eggplants until smooth.

2. Then mix up blended eggplants with garlic, egg, oatmeal, ground black pepper, and Parmesan. Make the small balls.

3. Heat the skillet with olive oil and put the eggplant balls inside. Roast them for on high heat for 1 minute per side.

Italian Style Eggplant Chips

Prep Time: 10 min

Cook Time: 5 min

Serve: 10

Ingredients:

- 2 eggplants, thinly sliced

- 1 tsp. ground black pepper

- 1 tsp. Italian seasonings

- 1 tbsp. olive oil

Preparation:

1. Rub the eggplant sliced with ground black pepper and Italian seasonings.

2. Then sprinkle the vegetable sliced with olive oil.

3. Grill the eggplant sliced for 2 minutes per side at 400F or until the vegetables are crunchy.

Lentil Dip

Prep Time: 10 min

Cook Time: 0 min

Serve: 7

Ingredients:

- 1 cup green lentils, cooked

- 1 tbsp. apple cider vinegar

- 1 tomato, chopped

- 1 tsp. olive oil

- 2 oz Parmesan, grated

Preparation:

Mix up all ingredients in the bowl and blend gently with the help of the immersion blender.

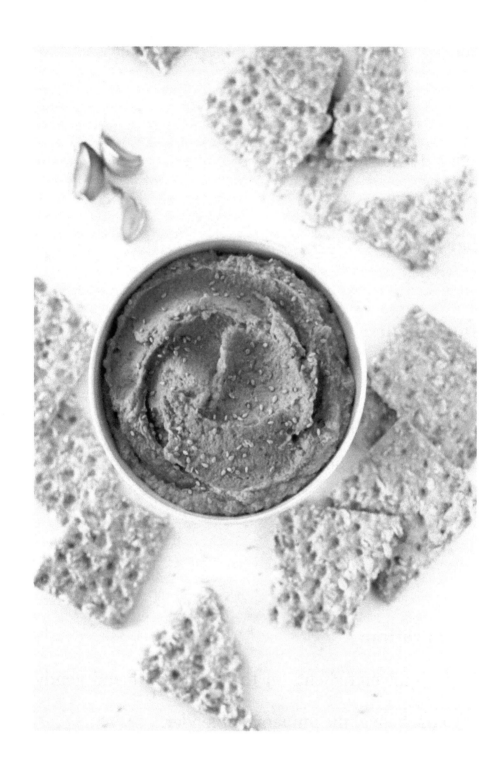

Delicious White Bean Hummus

Prep Time: 10 min

Cook Time: 25 min

Serve: 16

Ingredients:

- Roasted Tomatoes as needed

- 1 head of garlic

- 30 ounce cooked cannellini beans

- 1 tbsp lemon juice

- 1/2 tsp salt

Preparation:

1. Set the oven to 400 degrees F and let it preheat meanwhile remove the tip of the garlic head and loose papery coating. Get a 6-ounce custard cup and add garlic.

2. Drizzle with 1 tsp of oil and then cover it with foil. Place your custard into the heated oven and bake for 25 minutes until the garlic head is soft. When it is done uncover the custard cup let it cool and squeeze the garlic.

3. Place the garlic into a food processor and add the cannellini beans lemon juice oil and salt. Pulse until well blended. Tip the hummus into the bowl and drizzle with olive oil. Add roasted tomatoes and serve with some vegetables.

Delicious Greek Quesadillas

Prep Time: 20 min

Cook Time: 10 min

Serve: 8

Ingredients:

- 1/2 cup julienned sun dried tomatoes in olive oil drained
- 1/2 cup chopped pitted Kalamata olives
- 10-ounces of frozen chopped spinach thawed and drained
- cup shredded mozzarella cheese
- 1 cup crumbled feta cheese
- 8 flour tortillas about 8 inch each
- 1 tbsp fresh dill
- The Tzatziki sauce

- 1 cup Greek yoghurt

- 1 medium cucumber diced

- 1 tsp chopped fresh mint optional

- 1 tsp lemon zest

- 1 tbsp lemon juice

- 1 tbsp chopped fresh dill

- 1 tsp minced garlic

- 2 tbsp olive oil

- 1/2 tsp salt

- 1/2 tsp ground black pepper

Preparation:

1. Set your oven to 400 degrees F and let preheat. Meanwhile prepare your sauce. Place your cucumber in a bowl and add mint lemon zest and juice yoghurt black pepper garlic dill and salt until well incorporated.

2. Drizzle this with olive oil and let it chill for about 10 minutes in the refrigerator. Put tortilla in a clean space. Add your spinach tomatoes cheese and olives and then cover with another tortilla.

3. Repeat these steps for making a quesadillas 3 times in the same way and place them on a large baking sheet lined with a parchment sheet.

4. Place the baking sheet into the oven and let cook for 10 minutes until the cheese melts completely. Serve these quesadillas with your delicious tzatziki sauce.

Garlic with Escarole

Prep Time: 5 min

Cook Time: 7 min

Serves: 4

Ingredients:

- 1 and 1/2 tsp of garlic

- 1 head of escarole leaves torn

- 1/8 tsp red pepper flakes

- 1 and 1/2 tbsp olive oil

- 1 tsp salt

Preparation:

Place a medium skillet pan over medium high heat. Add garlic and cook for a couple of minutes until nicely golden brown. Stir in the red pepper flakes and add the escarole in batches. Season with salt and toss until it is well incorporated. Cook this for 5 minutes until the escarole leaves wilt. Serve immediately.

Cheddar Potato Crisps

Prep Time: 10 min

Cook Time: 0 min

Serve: 4

Ingredients:

- 1 cup Greek yogurt (unsweetened)

- 1/2 cup grated cheddar cheese

- 6 red potatoes, thinly sliced

- 1/2 cup chives

- 3 slices ham

- Cooking oil or spray as required

- Salt and black pepper to taste

Preparation:

1. Take the potatoes; sprinkle with salt and black pepper.

2. Cover and place in the refrigerator for 30 minutes. Heat a grill at medium temperature setting. Spray the potato slices with cooking oil, place over a baking sheet and grill for about 2 minutes.

3. Flip and grill for 2 more minutes. Add the ham slices to the baking sheet and grill for one minute.

4. Add the potato and ham in a serving bowl. Top with the chives, yogurt and grated cheese as desired.

Healthy Coconut Blueberry Balls

Prep Time: 10 min

Cook Time: 10 min

Serve: 12

Ingredients:

- ¼ cup flaked coconut

- ¼ cup blueberries

- ½ tsp. vanilla

- ¼ cup honey

- ½ cup creamy almond butter

- ¼ tsp. cinnamon

- 1 ½ tbsp. chia seeds

- ¼ cup flaxseed meal

- 1 cup rolled oats, gluten-free

Preparation:

1. In a large bowl, add oats, cinnamon, chia seeds, and flaxseed meal and mix well. Add almond butter in microwave-safe bowl and microwave for 30 seconds. Stir until smooth. Add vanilla and honey in melted almond butter and stir well.

2.. Pour almond butter mixture over oat mixture and stir to combine. Add coconut and blueberries and stir well.

3. Make small balls from oat mixture and place onto the baking tray and place in the refrigerator for 1 hour. Serve and enjoy.

Crunchy Roasted Chickpeas

Prep Time: 10 min

Cook Time: 25 min

Serve: 4

Ingredients:

- 15 oz can chickpeas, drained, rinsed and pat dry

- ¼ tsp. paprika

- 1 tbsp. olive oil

- ¼ tsp. pepper

- Pinch of salt

Preparation:

1. Preheat the oven to 450°F. Spray a baking tray with cooking spray and set aside.

2. In a large bowl, toss chickpeas with olive oil and spread chickpeas onto the prepared baking tray.

3. Roast chickpeas in preheated oven for 25 minutes. Shake after every 10 minutes. Once chickpeas are done then immediately toss with paprika, pepper, and salt.

Tasty Zucchini Chips

Prep Time: 10 min

Cook Time: 15 min

Serve: 8

Ingredients:

- 2 medium zucchini, sliced 4mm thick

- ½ tsp. paprika

- ¼ tsp. garlic powder

- ¾ cup parmesan cheese, grated

- 4 tbsp. olive oil

- ¼ tsp. pepper

- Pinch of salt

Preparation:

1. Preheat the oven to 375°F. Spray a baking tray with cooking spray and set aside. In a bowl, combine the oil, garlic powder, paprika, pepper, and salt.

2. Add sliced zucchini and toss to coat. Arrange zucchini slices onto the prepared baking tray and sprinkle grated cheese on top. Bake in preheated oven for 15 minutes or until lightly golden brown. Serve and enjoy.

Roasted Green Beans

Prep Time: 10 min

Cook Time: 15 min

Serve: 4

Ingredients:

- 1 lb green beans

- 4 tbsp. parmesan cheese

- 2 tbsp. olive oil

- ¼ tsp. garlic powder

- Pinch of salt

Preparation:

1. Preheat the oven to 400°F. Add green beans in a large bowl. Add remaining ingredients on top of green beans and toss to coat.

2. Spread green beans onto the baking tray and roast in preheated oven for 15 minutes. Stir halfway through.

3. Serve and enjoy.

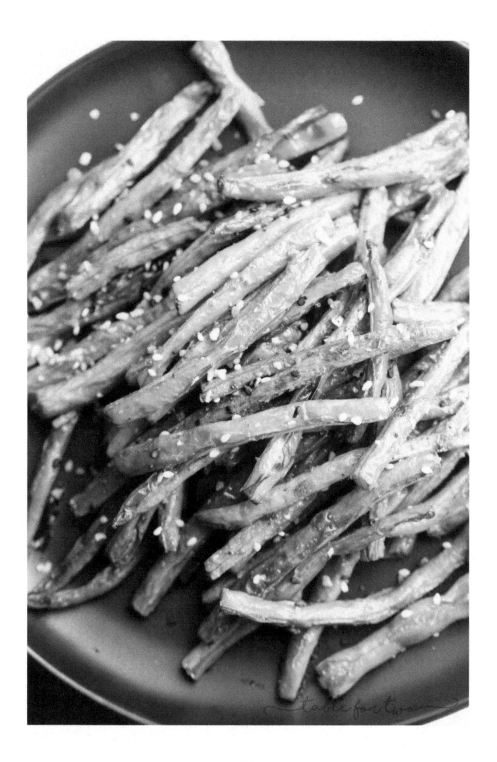

Savory Pistachio Balls

Prep Time: 10 min

Cook Time: 5 min

Serve: 16

Ingredients:

- ½ cup pistachios, unsalted
- 1 cup dates, pitted
- ½ tsp. ground fennel seeds
- ½ cup raisins
- Pinch of pepper

Preparation:

Add all ingredients into the food processor and process until well combined. Make small balls and place onto the baking tray and place in the refrigerator for 1 hour. Serve and enjoy.

Roasted Almonds

Prep Time: 10 min

Cook Time: 20 min

Serve: 12

Ingredients:

- 2 ½ cups almonds

- ¼ tsp. cayenne

- ¼ tsp. ground coriander

- ¼ tsp. cumin

- ¼ tsp. chili powder

- 1 tbsp. fresh rosemary, chopped

- 1 tbsp. olive oil

- 2 ½ tbsp. maple syrup

- Pinch of salt

Preparation:

1. Preheat the oven to 325°F. Spray a baking tray with cooking spray and set aside.

2. In a mixing bowl, whisk together oil, cayenne, coriander, cumin, chili powder, rosemary, maple syrup, and salt.

3. Add almond and stir to coat. Spread almonds onto the prepared baking tray. Roast almonds in preheated oven for 20 minutes. Stir halfway through. Serve and enjoy.

Banana Strawberry Popsicles

Prep Time: 5 min

Cook Time: 0 min

Serve: 8

Ingredients:

- ½ cup Greek yogurt
- 1 banana, peeled and sliced
- 1 ¼ cup fresh strawberries
- ¼ cup of water

Preparation:

1. Add all ingredients into the blender and blend until smooth. Pour blended mixture into the popsicles molds and place in the refrigerator for 4 hours or until set.

2. Serve and enjoy.

Chocolate Matcha Balls

Prep Time: 10 min

Cook Time: 5 min

Serve: 15

- 2 tbsp. unsweetened cocoa powder

- 3 tbsp. oats, gluten-free

- ½ cup pine nuts

- ½ cup almonds

- 1 cup dates, pitted

- 2 tbsp. matcha powder

Preparation:

1. Add oats, pine nuts, almonds, and dates into a food processor and process until well combined. Place matcha powder in a small dish.

2. Make small balls from mixture and coat with matcha powder. Enjoy or store in refrigerator until ready to eat.

Chia Almond Butter Pudding

Prep Time: 5 min

Cook Time: 5 min

Serve: 1

Ingredients:

- ¼ cup chia seeds

- 1 cup unsweetened almond milk

- 1 ½ tbsp. maple syrup

- 2 ½ tbsp. almond butter

Preparation:

1. Add almond milk, maple syrup, and almond butter in a bowl and stir well. Add chia seeds and stir to mix.

2. Pour pudding mixture into the Mason jar and place in the refrigerator for overnight. Serve and enjoy.

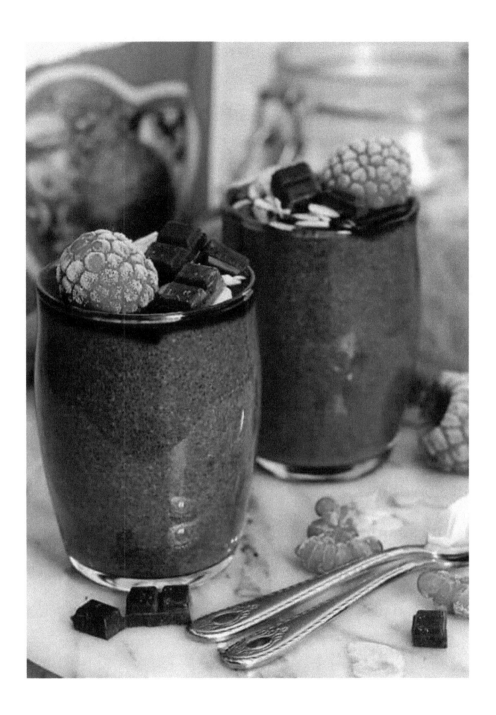

Refreshing Strawberry

Popsicles

Prep Time: 5 min

Cook Time: 5 min

Serve: 8

Ingredients:

- ½ cup almond milk

- 2 ½ cup fresh strawberries

Preparation:

1. Add strawberries and almond milk into the blender and blend until smooth. Pour strawberry mixture into popsicles molds and place in the refrigerator for 4 hours or until set.

2. Serve and enjoy.

Dark Chocolate Mousse

Prep Time: 10 min

Cook Time: 10 min

Serve: 4

Ingredients:

- 3.50z unsweetened dark chocolate, grated

- ½ tsp. vanilla

- 1 tbsp. honey

- 2 cups Greek yogurt

- ¾ cup unsweetened almond milk

Preparation:

1. Add chocolate and almond milk in a saucepan and heat over medium heat until just chocolate melted. Do not boil.

2. Once the chocolate and almond milk combined then add vanilla and honey and stir well. Add yogurt in a large mixing bowl. Pour chocolate mixture on top of yogurt and mix until well combined.

3. Pour chocolate yogurt mixture into the serving bowls and place in refrigerator for 2 hours. Top with fresh raspberries.

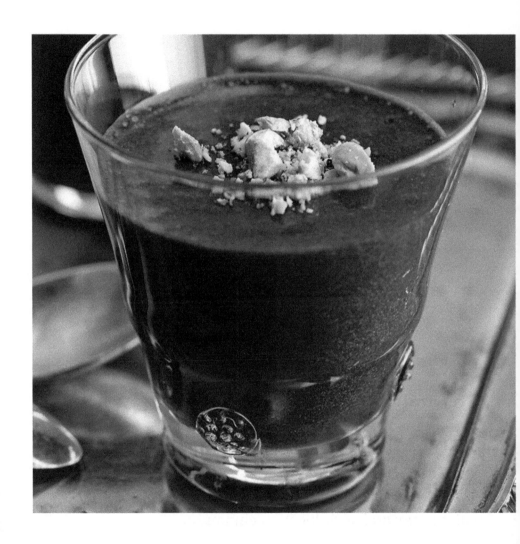

Warm & Soft Baked Pears

Prep Time: 10 min

Cook Time: 25 min

Serve: 4

Ingredients:

- 4 pears, cut in half and core
- ½ tsp. vanilla
- ¼ tsp. cinnamon
- ½ cup maple syrup

Preparation:

1. Preheat the oven to 375°F. Spray a baking tray with cooking spray. Arrange pears, cut side up on a prepared baking tray and sprinkle with cinnamon.

2. In a small bowl, whisk vanilla and maple syrup and drizzle over pears. Bake pears in preheated oven for 25 minutes. Serve and enjoy.

Healthy & Quick Energy Bites

Prep Time: 10 min

Cook Time: 0 min

Serve: 20

Ingredients:

- 2 cups cashew nuts

- ¼ tsp. cinnamon

- 1 tsp. lemon zest

- 4 tbsp. dates, chopped

- 1/3 cup unsweetened shredded coconut

- ¾ cup dried apricots

Preparation:

1. Line baking tray with parchment paper and set aside.

2. Add all ingredients in a food processor and process until the mixture is crumbly and well combined. Make small balls from mixture and place on a prepared baking tray.

3. Place in refrigerator for 1 hour. Serve and enjoy.

Creamy Yogurt Banana Bowls

Prep Time: 10 min

Cook Time: 0 min

Serve: 4

Ingredients:

- 2 bananas, sliced

- ½ tsp. ground nutmeg

- 3 tbsp. flaxseed meal

- ¼ cup creamy peanut butter

- 4 cups Greek yogurt

Preparation:

1. Divide Greek yogurt between 4 serving bowls and top with sliced bananas. Add peanut butter in microwave-safe bowl and microwave for 30 seconds.

2. Drizzle 1 tbsp. of melted peanut butter on each bowl on top of the sliced bananas.

3. Sprinkle cinnamon and flax meal on top and serve.

Chicken Wings Platter

Prep Time: 10 min

Cook Time: 20 min

Serve: 4

Ingredients:

- 2 lb. chicken wings

- ½ cup tomato sauce

- A pinch of salt and black pepper

- 1 tsp. smoked paprika

- 1 tbsp. cilantro, chopped

- 1 tbsp. chives, chopped

Preparation:

1. In your instant pot, combine the chicken wings with the sauce and the rest of the ingredients, stir, put the lid on and cook on High for 20 minutes.

2. Release the pressure naturally for 10 minutes, arrange the chicken wings on a platter and serve as an appetizer.

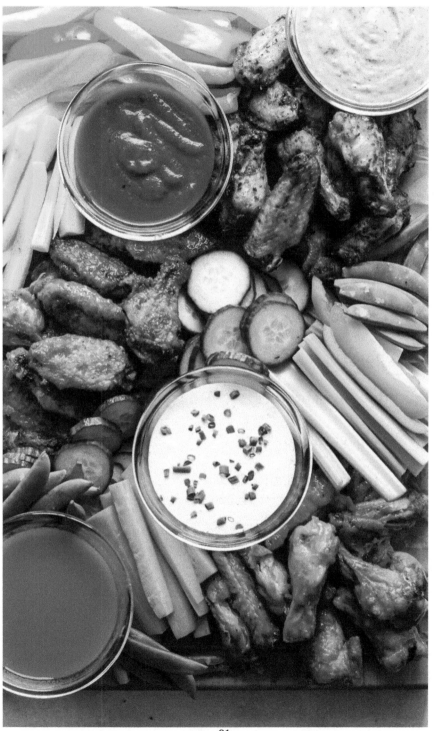

Carrot Spread

Prep Time: 10 min

Cook Time: 10 min

Serve: 4

Ingredients:

- ¼ cup veggie stock

- A pinch of salt and black pepper

- 1 tsp. onion powder

- ½ tsp. garlic powder

- ½ tsp. oregano, dried

- 1 lb. carrots, sliced

- ½ cup coconut cream

Preparation:

1. In your instant pot, combine all the ingredients except the cream, put the lid on and cook on High for 10 minutes.

2. Release the pressure naturally for 10 minutes, transfer the carrots mix to food processor, add the cream, pulse well, divide into bowls and serve cold.

Chocolate Mousse

Prep Time: 10 min

Cook Time: 6 min

Serve: 5

Ingredients:

- 4 egg yolks

- ½ tsp. vanilla

- ½ cup unsweetened almond milk

- 1 cup whipping cream

- ¼ cup cocoa powder

- ¼ cup water

- ½ cup Swerve

- 1/8 tsp. salt

Preparation:

1. Add egg yolks to a large bowl and whisk until well beaten.

2. In a saucepan, add swerve, cocoa powder, and water and whisk until well combined. Add almond milk and cream to the saucepan and whisk until well mix.

3. Once saucepan mixtures are heated up then turn off the heat. Add vanilla and salt and stir well.

4. Add a tbsp. of chocolate mixture into the eggs and whisk until well combined. Slowly pour remaining chocolate to the eggs and whisk until well combined.

5. Pour batter into the ramekins. Pour 1 ½ cups of water into the instant pot then place a trivet in the pot. Place ramekins on a trivet. Seal pot with lid and select manual and set timer for 6 minutes. Release pressure using quick release method than open the lid.

6. Carefully remove ramekins from the instant pot and let them cool completely. Serve and enjoy.

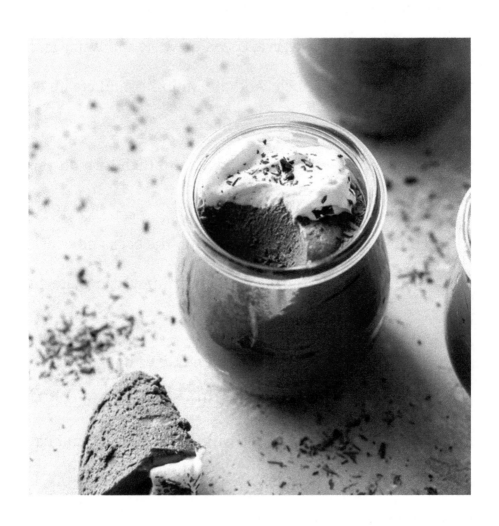

Veggie Fritters

Prep Time: 10 min

Cook Time: 10 min

Serve: 4

Ingredients:

- 2 garlic cloves, minced
- 2 yellow onions, chopped
- 4 scallions, chopped
- 2 carrots, grated
- 2 tsp. cumin, ground
- ½ tsp. turmeric powder
- Salt and black pepper to the taste
- ¼ tsp. coriander, ground
- 2 tbsp. parsley, chopped
- ¼ tsp. lemon juice

- ½ cup almond flour

- 2 beets, peeled and grated

- 2 eggs, whisked

- ¼ cup tapioca flour

- 3 tbsp. olive oil

Preparation:

1. In a bowl, combine the garlic with the onions, scallions and the rest of the ingredients except the oil, stir well and shape medium patties out of this mix.

2. Heat a pan with the oil over medium-high heat, add the patties, cook for 5 minutes on each side, arrange on a platter and serve.

White Bean Dip

Prep Time: 10 min

Cook Time: 0 min

Serve: 4

Ingredients:

- 15 oz. canned white beans, drained and rinsed
- 6 oz. canned artichoke hearts, drained and quartered
- 4 garlic cloves, minced
- 1 tbsp. basil, chopped
- 2 tbsp. olive oil
- Juice of ½ lemon
- Zest of ½ lemon, grated
- Salt and black pepper to the taste

Preparation:

In your food processor, combine the beans with the artichokes and the rest of the ingredients except the oil and pulse well. Add the oil gradually, pulse the mix again, divide into cups and serve as a party dip.

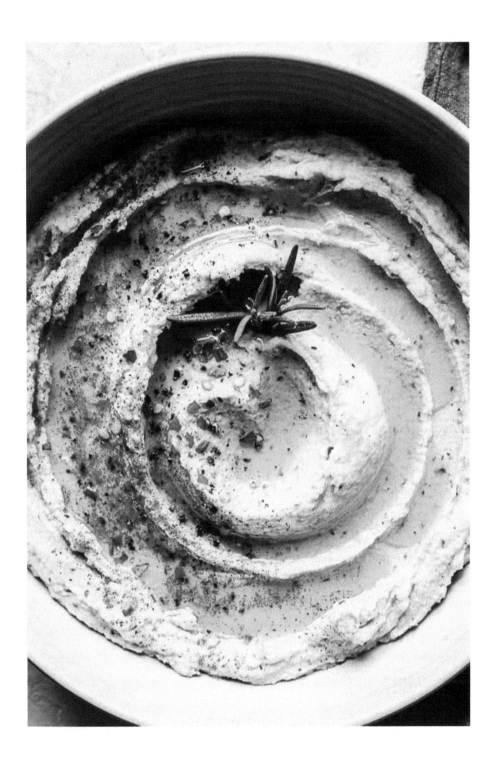

Stuffed Sweet Potato

Prep Time: 10 min

Cook Time: 40 min

Serve: 8

Ingredients:

- 8 sweet potatoes, pierced with a fork
- 14 oz. canned chickpeas, drained and rinsed
- 1 small red bell pepper, chopped
- 1 tbsp. lemon zest, grated
- 2 tbsp. lemon juice
- 3 tbsp. olive oil
- 1 tsp. garlic, minced
- 1 tbsp. oregano, chopped
- 2 tbsp. parsley, chopped
- A pinch of salt and black pepper

- 1 avocado, peeled, pitted and mashed

- ¼ cup water

- ¼ cup tahini paste

Preparation:

1. Arrange the potatoes on a baking sheet lined with parchment paper, bake them at 400°F for 40 minutes, cool them down and cut a slit down the middle in each.

2. In a bowl, combine the chickpeas with the bell pepper, lemon zest, half of the lemon juice, half of the oil, half of the garlic, oregano, half of the parsley, salt and pepper, toss and stuff the potatoes with this mix.

3. In another bowl, mix the avocado with the water, tahini, the rest of the lemon juice, oil, garlic and parsley, whisk well and spread over the potatoes. Serve cold for breakfast.

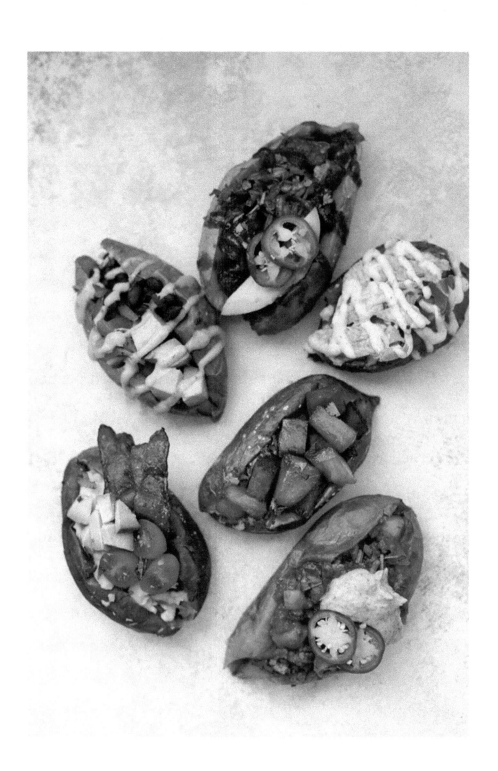

Rosemary Bulgur Appetizer

Prep Time: 25 min

Cook Time: 0 min

Serve: 6

Ingredients:

- ½ cup couscous

- 2 tbsp. olive oil

- 1 ¾ cup onions, chopped

- 2 cups vegetable broth

- 1 cup bulgur

- 1 tbsp. chives, chopped

- 1 tbsp. parsley, chopped

- ¼ tsp. rosemary, chopped

Preparation:

1. Over medium stove flame; heat the oil in a skillet or saucepan (preferably medium size). Sauté the onions until softened and translucent, stir in between.

2. Add the bulgur and 1 ½ cups vegetable broth; simmer the mixture until the bulgur is tender.

3. Remove it from the heat and fluff with a fork. In another skillet or saucepan, heat the remaining vegetable broth and simmer. Add the oil and couscous. Stir and cook this until your couscous is tender. Fluff it with a fork.

4. In a mixing bowl, combine the bulgur and couscous. Add the rosemary, chives and parsley on top. Season it with black pepper and salt. Serve as an appetizer or light meal

Lightning Source UK Ltd.
Milton Keynes UK
UKHW020657140521
383710UK00001B/31